DMSO

THE UNIVERSAL HEALING WONDER DRUG.

BY

DR. CHERRY ARMSTRONG.

Copyright 2022. All rights Reserved

<u>**foreword.**</u>

...this book is a must-read for anyone and everyone who wants to learn (on an educational basis), medical research, and practical administration (but under the strict supervision) of a qualified health practitioner as duly spelled out by the author on the back cover page of this book. You will like it!

... Dr. Gideon Rich (Louisa Medical Outreach)

Table of Contents.

CHAPTER ONE.

INTRODUCTION.

DMSO (Dimethylsulfoxide) is a prescriptive medicinal drug and dietary supplement. It can be taken orally (via the mouth), rubbed on the pores and skin (used topically), or injected into the veins (intravenously).

DMSO is taken orally, topically, or intravenously in other to manage Amyloidosis and other related ailments. Amyloidosis is simply a situation in which certain proteins are abnormally deposited in vital organs and tissues of the body system.

This therapeutic drug is used topically to decrease aches and enhance wound recovery, muscle aches, burns, and other skeletal injuries. Topical application of DMSO also helps deal with painful conditions like headache, irritation, osteoarthritis, rheumatoid arthritis, and severe facial ache known as tic-douloureux. It's occasionally used for eye conditions like cataracts, glaucoma, and retina issues; for foot conditions like fungi on toe-nails, calluses, and bunions, calluses; for pores and skin conditions such as keloid scars alongside scleroderma. DMSO is sometimes used to deal with damage to skin and tissues due to leakage from chemotherapy IV. DMSO therapy can be used either on its own or mixed with idoxuridine to treat shingles (herpes zoster-related infections).

DMSO is used intravenously to reduce abnormal blood pressure within the brain and to address bladder infections like interstitial cystitis and persistent inflammatory bladder diseases.

This alternative medicine (DMSO) possesses an in-depth spectrum of pharmacological results, such as local analgesia, membrane piercing/penetration, susceptible bacteriostasis, and anti-inflammatory functions.

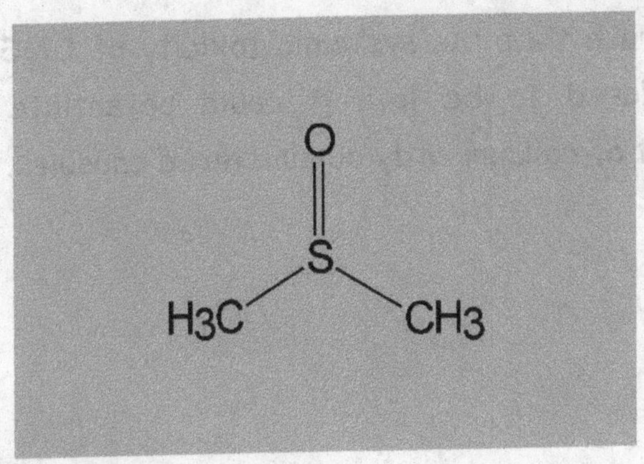

The essential use of DMSO is as a medium of transporting different drugs around the body, thereby enhancing the effectiveness of those drugs and supporting the penetration of various pills into the skin. It is also used as a cryo-protectant for various human tissues.

The efficacy and protection of DMSO are especially uncertain; few studies have been carried out to allow for conclusions on its use dependably. It penetrates faster via the tissues, and there aren't any outstanding variations among its consequences after one-of-a-type routes of administration. However, the reactions are uncommon but can be averted substantially through the use of more dilute solutions. Despite the truth that the systemic toxicity of DMSO is considered to be low, it could potentiate the effect of concurrently administered capsules.

CHAPTER TWO.
DEFINITION OF DMSO.

DMSO also known as dimethyl sulfoxide is simply a colorless oily fluid derived from trees as a by-product of the paper production process. Its crystalline by-product called MSM (methylsulfonyl methane) shares nearly equal traits as DMSO except that it does not produce the garlic-like breath and body odor commonly visible with DMSO usage.

DMSO is commonly used as an industrial solvent as well as a paint cleanser. It is seen as the most efficient solution for symptomatic treatments of continual genitourinary issues alongside trigonitis, prostatitis, interstitial cystitis, cystitis, and radiation cystitis.

DMSO is likewise authorized to be used as a preservative for bone marrow and stem cells which might be saved for further use. In extraordinarily lively populations in addition to athletes and army personnel, DMSO is well-known

13

as a remedy for musculoskeletal injuries as well as reduces pains related to a few musculoskeletal injuries.

ORIGINATION OF DMSO.

DMSO came into existence in 1866 at the Volga River through the discovery of a Russian scientist known as Alexander Saytzeff in Kazan, Central Russia. He observed that the substance was colorless, felt oily when touched, seems like mineral oil when poured into a test tube with a taste like that of clams or oysters, and had a garlic-like odor. It works well as an oil or paint remover, and also as an anti-freeze. From his discovery, pharmacists began to develop an interest in this substance at end of the 2nd World War. By 1948, DMSO was seen in various published papers as an excellent solvent.

In 1959, some British crew validated the protective ability of DMSO on red blood cells and other vital tissues from cold. It has a high eventuality for dissolving substances. It's a reagent that is suitable for speeding up chemical responses by billions of reiterations. The unique capability of DMSO to pierce any living tissue without causing significant damage is most presumably due to its cool nature, its capacity to absorb hydrogen bonds, as well as its compact structure. As a result of these composites, DMSO can synthesize nucleic acids, ionic substances, water, carbohydrates, proteins, and other rudiments of the living system.

The capability of DMSO to modify other water motes associated with cellular factors or to intrude with the conformation of ubiquitous water is central to our understanding of its implicit functions in natural systems.

DMSO is a by-product of lignin and a sticky ingredient of trees in the United States. It can be mixed with coal, petroleum, or other organic material. The collective works of Jacob's staff from the University of Oregon Medical School and that of Herschler from Crown Zellerbach

Corporation through laboratory tests revealed that DMSO not only passes through the skin and mucous membranes but also carries several other factors. i.e Penicillin can be dissolved into DMSO and applied directly to the skin without the use of any needle material.

DMSO is a good solution for the relief of pain, preventing bacteria development/growth, softening red blood cells, reducing inflammation, enhancing the effectiveness of other pharmacologic agents, acting as a diuretic, and also relax other muscle tissues. It helps relieve cramps, pain, arthritis, and pains from broken bones. Veterinarians use DMSO _for_ animal-related injuries like arthritic conditions.

CHAPTER THREE

HOW DMSO WORKS.

DMSO aids other medications to get through the skin and positively impacts water, carbohydrates fats, and protein flow in the body frame. It is effective for treating ailments such as:

- Headaches.

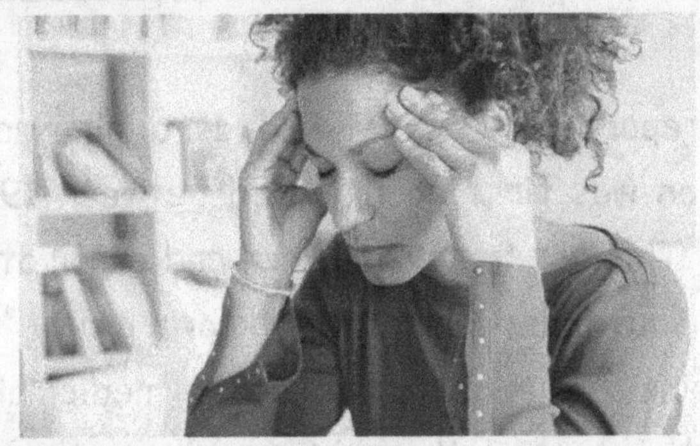

- Asthma.
- Muscle problems.
- Cancer.
- Bladder disease: Bladder inflammation (interstitial cystitis).
- Skin and tissue damage from leaked IV chemotherapy.

- Shingles (herpes zoster infection).
- Eye problems.
- Foot ulcers caused by diabetes.
- Scleroderma.
- High blood pressure to the brain system.
- Arthritis.
- Amyloidosis and several other health conditions.

CONTROVERSIES SURROUNDING DMSO ORIGIN.

The report on DMSO used as a pharmacologic solution was first documented between 1963 and 1964. This led to several trial and error attempts by various individuals having known a new "wonder medicine" that can drive other medicinal drugs into the pores of the skin as well as other organs of the body, and eliminate pains and inflammations in the same vein.

The FDA (Food and Drug Agency) granted the first Investigational New Drug (IND) petition for DMSO clinical testing in humans on October 25, 1963. With time, this medicinal agent gained widespread acceptance as a treatment for small burns, abrasions, and acne. The medicine is given away without charge by a huge number of general medical investigators, specialists, and first aid experts, including physiotherapists, a few dentists, nurses, and other medical practitioners.

There erupt some disagreements about the use of DMSO when some scientists became interested in how they can securely freeze human kidneys using DMSO as a solution. Since DMSO is a by-product of the paper-making process, he requested more DMSO chemicals from paper-producing companies.

It was noted that the drying effect of DMSO causes explosion and moisture frequently fosters infection, hence a drying agent is helpful in the treatment of burns and DMSO became a possible solution for such effect. Further research on burned mice revealed that those who got treated with DMSO solution had moral calmness compared to those who did not. The drug helped lessen the burning sensation.

It was estimated that about 100,000 patients had already been treated using DMSO therapy as of the year 1965. But the FDA did not accept these results as accurate irrespective of the research that has been done because they felt that the benefits might not be related to DMSO medication. The closest thing to a "great medicine", according to the New York Times, is DMSO. The FDA, however, rejected it and republished its statement outlining all clinical uses of DMSO in the Federal Register.

It was discovered that large doses of this medicine hurt the ocular lenses of test animals in toxicological experiments. That is, the lenses had some clouds on them and their ability to focus had changed.

The Orgnisation, therefore, had a personal stake in persons exposed to DMSO suffering the clear potential harm. Although it wasn't known to academics and authorities at the time that only a few species exposed to this agent has eye changes, both the monkeys and, more crucially, the humans who were tested with this medicine experienced no negative side effects. The FDA allowed a new clinical trial of DMSO in patients with serious illnesses like advanced herpes zoster infection, severe rheumatoid arthritis, and scleroderma for which there is no effective treatment a year after the ban policy was partially loosened.

A further revision was made by the FDA in September 1968 to relax their previous policy regarding the ban on DMSO usage. This new policy allowed DMSO to be used only for 14 days on the skin to prevent any negative adverse effects. The policy review came as a result of further toxicological studies on humans that gave a re-assurance that there were no toxic effects in humans after the experiment.

PUBLIC VIEWS ABOUT THE FOOD AND DRUG AGENCY'S POLICY ON DMSO.

DMSO as an alternative medicine remained available to most Americans irrespective of the ban placed on its use by the FDA. It became business for some, whilst others are looking for DMSO remedies at the orthopedic clinics in Mexico as it passes from person to person, especially amongst arthritis patients.

The two fundamental health issues dealt with using DMSO human exponents were osteoarthritis and rheumatoid arthritis. It became surprising to people why rubbing DMSO solution on the skin is not safe when it is a safe remedy for treating internal interstitial cystitis.

The alternative market place for the delivery of this alternative medicine has been improved upon, it is being prescribed by medical practitioners.

CHAPTER FOUR.

DMSO'S TOXICITY AND POSSIBLE SIDE EFFECTS.

DMSO is not harmful at all as it was stipulated. It's no longer true that anything is dangerous about this medication. Aspirin is far less safe than DMSO as a medication. People die after taking aspirin, but no death has been recorded from the use of DMSO. Numerous controlled studies have shown that it is both strong and safe for use.

LABORATORY EXPERIMENT OUTCOME ON ANIMAL DMSO TOXICITY.

The conclusion reached by scientists that have made their research about DMSO using 8 species of mammals, including humans, along with a few fish and birds, is that it has low toxicity. Many animals have been given this medication both for a short- and long-term period, and it has been discovered that they tolerate it so well. When given to, injected into, or applied to the skin of human and animal research subjects for weeks, months, or years, there were either no or little signs or symptoms of any toxic reaction. People require the painkiller effect that DMSO offers and claim that even if there are slight side effects, they are worth it, given the benefits this medication offers (the benefit outweighs the side effect). Because DMSO dissolves a wide variety of materials and can be absorbed via the skin, combining solvent and other different compounds have been researched as well. Some chemicals' toxicity or their rate of absorption changes after being dissolved in DMSO while some remain the same.

Simply put, DMSO enhances their healing capacity. Technologically, the toxicity of a substance is determined by its LD (Lethal dose), which is the amount of DMSO in milligrams(mg) per kilogram(kg) of the test animal's body weight that results in the possible death of half the animals being tested. The average observation period is between 1-4 weeks period. Consequently, 100 guinea pigs can get DMSO for 1-2 weeks at a dosage of 2mg per 0.45kg (1 pound), resulting in a dose of roughly 3mg dose of DMSO for a 3-pounds of guinea pig.

By increasing this dosage (lethal dose/LD_{50}) to half, the animals perish at the same time hence pointing to the toxic effect. Calculating the healing index involves dividing the poisonous dose by the healing dose. This healing index provides information to researchers and doctors on the toxicity of a drug or other substance to living things, particularly people.

The safer the medicine, the higher the healing index quantity. It is poisonous if there is a minor variation in the healing index. Unlike Aspirin which has an LD_{50} of 558mg/kg in monkeys when consumed, DMSO has an LD_{50} of 4,000mg/kg in monkeys. Therefore, DMSO is seven times safer than aspirin. According to studies done on laboratory mice's skin, the LD_{50} for DMSO has been calculated to be 50,000mg/kg and they can withstand complete immersion in up to 60% of DMSO solution.

Rats can survive an 80% DMSO dipping as well as a repeated dipping of about 60% quantity for at least 21 days to 4 months, which is the LD_{50} of a

DMSO's single-dose toxicity. The application of DMSO to human skin normally causes some reddening, but the effect is frequently not significant after repeated applications. Thirty-five percent (35%) of those who use the substance claim that it gives them a burning sensation when they touch something. Lesser numbers of people report light irritation, skin roughness, thickening, blistering, and dermatitis. However, these are just minor effects rather than toxic reactions. Dryness or the skin's natural process of removing fat is one major cause of these effects in most cases. Most often, odors can be sensed in the skin's pores and breath. Toxic effects from the medication could result from inhalation. As DMSO's vapor strain is about 0.6mm/Hg at 77°F, it evaporates slowly. As a result, when applied to the skin, the awareness of DMSO in the air may, in most instances, be very minimal. The user should exercise the same caution against inhalation when heated or sprayed as they would with any natural solvent.

Depending on the application method and level of awareness, adding DMSO to blood might result in a variety of effects. There are no cancer-causing properties in DMSO. Additionally, the medication is no longer sold for hypersensitive reactions. The use of DMSO doesn't worsen common hypersensitive reactions in people, such as those brought on by house dust, pet hair, combined grasses, or weeds. Be aware, though, that some people's skin inflammation brought on by a solvent may also encourage the growth of some allergens, the substances that trigger an allergic reaction. When DMSO is administered in any method, it first absorbs and penetrates the bloodstream through the circulatory system of the skin where it circulates tissues all over the body. A study on cats found that 3% of DMSO is expelled inside the breath as dimethyl sulfide, and some of it is metabolized to dimethyl sulfone. *The dimethyl-sulfide derivative produced by the body's metabolic process is what causes DMSO patients' breath to smell bad.* Such metabolized products aren't harmful in the quantifiable amounts found inside the body. It is also important to remember that asparagus, cooked maize, coffee, tea, milk, clams, and tomatoes all contain dimethyl sulfide, which is a major causative factor of halitosis (bad breath). The use of DMSO has certain undesirable side effects, but none are dangerous. The superior blessings appear to be far more than the undesirable side effect that comes with them.

<u>CHAPTER FIVE.</u>

<u>DMSO THERAPEUTICAL PRINCIPLE.</u>

This chapter looks into how DMSO works and talks about the purpose of its use as well as its penetration power. We shall try to make some complex biological theories as simple as we can without changing the theories that support DMSO activities.

<u>DMSO'S MOLECULAR STRUCTURE AND PHYSICAL CONDITIONS.</u>

* The heart of the ten-sided dimethylsulfoxide molecule contains an atom of sulfur. Methyl groups, an oxygen atom, and a non-binding electron pair make up the tetrahedron's components.
* DMSO has a molecular weight of 78.15.
* The drug releases 60 calories per gram (g) of DMSO when combined with water, causing a chemical reaction that results in the internal formation of heat.

♣ At 76.0 mm of mercury (Hg), the boiling factor is 189.0 degrees Celsius (°C).

♣ At 20 degrees Celsius, the vapor pressure is zero.37 mm Hg, while at 25 degrees Celsius, the specific gravity is 1.0958 g/ml.

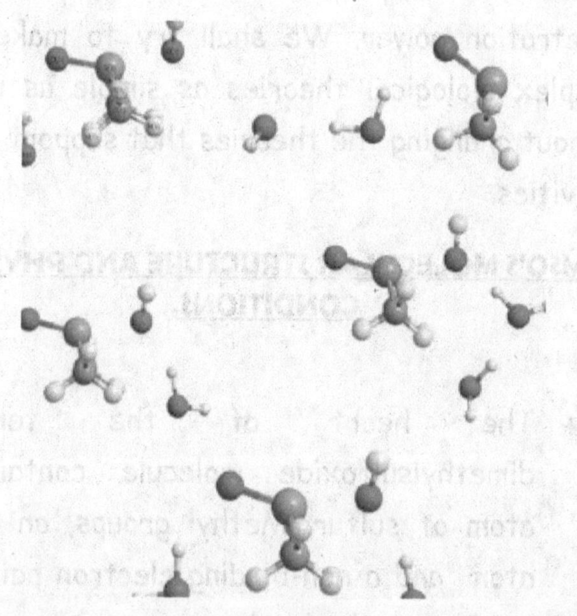

♣ The melting point is 18.55 °C, the warmth of combustion is 6.050 cal/g, and the flash point in an open vessel is 95 °C.

♣ At 20 degrees Celsius, the viscosity in centipoise (CP) is 2.473, and the floor anxiety in dynes per centimeter (cm) is 46.2. If a bottle of the liquid solvent is obtained from an unidentified source, its approximate concentration can be determined by DMSO's freezing factor of 68°F.

* Put the unopened bottle inside the refrigerator (not the freezer part). Ice will form out of the liquid in a few hours. You currently have 99.5% DMSO, which is the cleanest and most concentrated solution available.

* Liquid can freeze at 68°F or lower by preventing hydrolysis (decomposition) by leaving the bottle cap on.

* If water drips appear on the ice when the frozen bottle is turned upside down, the DMSO is most likely of a veterinary grade. This amounts to 90% of your attention. 10% of the entire debt is related to distilled water.

* If the DMSO does not freeze while being stored in the refrigerator and does not

solidify after being stored at temperatures below 32°F, it most likely contains a 50/50 mixture of DMSO and water. Place the DMSO in the freezer compartment.

* If it freezes (solidifies), it is either not DMSO or it is almost all water with a trace of DMSO quantity mixed in. A 50% concentration of DMSO acts as an anti-freeze and keeps engines running smoothly all winter.

* Place the hardened DMSO within the bottle in a pan of hot water to re-liquefy it. The solvent can live an infinite number of lives in its original form. DMSO has a long shelf life.

* In liquid form, DMSO appears to have a chain-like shape that is held together by the alignment of the two sulfur-oxygen poles. Due to the fact that many liquid properties, such as density, viscosity, or refractive index, exhibit dramatic changes in temperature coefficients in this temperature range, this shape is thought to

partially degrade between 40°C and 60°C. It's notable to medical practitioners that DMSO works well with molecules that have a lot of hydrogen ions on them as well as with neutral molecules and ionic species. Because of this, DMSO is seen as an excellent solvent that can pass across many inorganic and natural materials.

* In proportion to a substance's polarizing capacity, DMSO interacts more with certain materials. This type of molecular interaction encourages a drug's solubility in DMSO, but it is also wanted by the degree of a substance or an object's usable working power.

CHAPTER SIX.

THE HEALING PROPERTIES OF DMSO.

The underlying healing tenet of DMSO is that it can cause cell damage by altering the shape of the water inside the cell. Due to DMSO, mobile membrane permeability changes the typical flow of substances in and out of the cells.

DMSO is one unique nutrient that supports the development of white blood cells and prolonged immunological production of the Macrophage Migration Inhibitory Factor (MMIF is a type of natural chemotherapy that is continuously offered inside the frame). Macrophages (a large wandering white blood cells) eat and destroy foreign proteins found in the blood and tissues, including microorganisms and other cells. As a result, DMSO increases the immune system's efficacy by enabling macrophages to move through tissues more quickly.

Allergies are lessened by DMSO because it opens up the cell membrane and increases the number of cellular receptor sites available for attachment via specific antigens, the substances that trigger the body to produce antibodies. When antigens are detected in the blood or tissue, antibodies that have already been made or are naturally present respond to neutralize the antigens.

In addition to preventing the spread of cancer, this method aids in the development of immunity to infectious diseases. Sclerosis, ulcerative colitis, lepromatous leprosy, sarcoidosis, rheumatoid arthritis, most malignancies, lymphoid thyroiditis, and congenital illnesses linked to T-cell depletion or malfunction are among the diseases known to be connected to a reduction in mobile-mediated responses and immunity that is mediated by cells is frequently potentiated by DMSO.

Other properties of DMSO include, but are not limited to:

- DMSO is a straightforward, tiny molecule with exceptional chemical, biological, and physical properties. It has this "exothermic" property that is well-known to everyone.

- While DMSO is being diluted with water, heat is generated.

- DMSO neutralizes risk associated with Hydroxyl radicals (OH), a tiny time bomb with the capacity to blow up one's cell system.

- When hydroxyl radical and DMSO react, a chemical compound is created that is expelled from the kidney into the urine. No matter the severity of the illness, the production of "free radicals" such as hydroxyl, chloride, and others is a major problem in the disease process. This is one of the main reasons why the "free radical scavenger" DMSO is effective in treating a wide range of diseases, including arteriosclerosis, arthritis, and most malignancies.

- Since DMSO substitutes water in living cells, it has the wonderful property of healing sick cells by squelching free radicals there.

- Additionally, DMSO will make cell membranes more permeable, allowing contaminants to escape from the cell.

- Through a variety of intricate ways, DMSO decreases hypersensitive reflexes while increasing the frame's resilience to contamination.

Once DMSO substitutes water in the living cells, it kicks the wonderful process of healing sick cells by aiding fluid free access to these.

Additionally, DMSO will make cell membrane less permeable, allowing contaminants to

CHAPTER SEVEN.

DMSO APPLICATION.

The DMSO chemical is typically applied to the skin in the form of a liquid or a gel; the liquid is more potent, but people seem to prefer the gel type. Rather than rub it on the skin, people now coat/tap it on the skin.

All you have to do to get it to absorb is skillfully rub it into your skin for about 20-60 minutes before it dries up. Although it might not dry out completely, however, you can easily wipe off any excess. To get the most beneficial effect, a quantity ranging from 50% to 80%, and even 90% with caution is required.

On a general note, only a 50% concentration of DMSO should be applied to the face and neck region because they are more the face and neck should only use DMSO at a concentration of 50% because they are more vulnerable compared to other parts of the body. Topical usage of DMSO doses should be below 70% concentration in regions with decreased circulation. To develop skin tolerance, it is advisable to start with lower concentrations.

Check for skin sensitivity before moving on to the higher concentration. Treatment for some uncommon disorders, such as scleroderma or Peroni's disease (where plaques or features of thick fibrous tissue wrap the penis, thereby producing deformity and uncomfortable erections), can last for longer than a year. The individual clinical issue and the doctor's discretion will determine how frequently you should inject this solution.

Despite its bacteriostatic properties, antibiotics must be taken if the solvent is used for extended periods in areas with a reduced blood supply. The most common fitness difficulties for which people use topical DMSO at home are likely acute musculoskeletal injuries and inflammations. The more quickly the medicine is administered to the damaged area, the more potent the result.

Note: **The skin must be clean, dry, and unbroken for any topical application of the medication, not just for musculoskeletal issues. Sweat or excessive skin oil must be eliminated. Make sure that no pesticides or heavy metals were left to dry on the skin.**

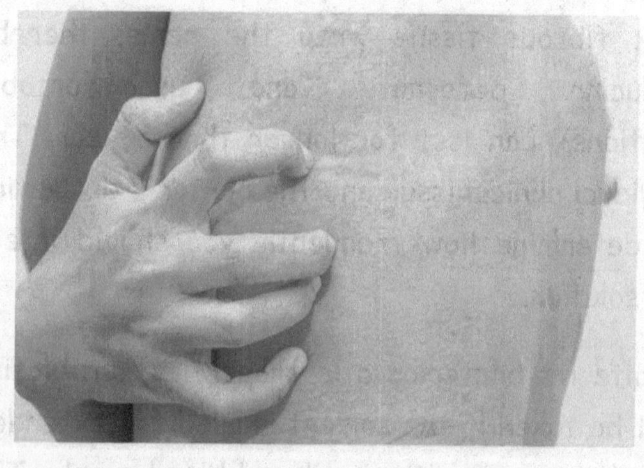

The clinical conditions that respond well are acute post-disturbing soft tissue injuries to the neck, shoulders, and back, sprains and lines of the larger joints of the top and lower limbs, acute post-worrying soft tissue injuries associated with intravenous and intramuscular hemorrhage regarding the trunks or the limbs, and acute bursitis regarding the major joints of the body.

For 4 out of 5 people, a 70% DMSO solution mixed with water in proportions ranging from 6-12ml, applied on and around the injury spot at least three times per day, would produce a potent recovery reaction with some relief within twenty-four hours.

For example, you can apply about 6ml of DMSO solution to the toe and the entire forefoot to treat gout of the large toe. Usually, it can take several minutes of repeated rubbing of this solution before an appropriate dosage can be obtained.

Allow the treated area to be exposed for 30-40 minutes; any remaining solution must then be removed using an absorbent cloth to prevent damage to your clothing. Within 30 minutes, gouty swelling and pain subside, lasting one to four hours. Repeated exercises up to four times per day will successfully alleviate acute gout pain.

There is consistently a high propensity for it to cause itching, redness, warmth, and irritations when a concentration of roughly 60-90% of DMSO is applied directly to the skin. This local inflammation often disappears in three hours.

Skin surfaces around the elbow and knee joints, as well as those on the face, neck, and armpits, are sensitive to a high concentration of DMSO solution. The skin may also wrinkle and continue to wrinkle for several days when a 60-90% solution is applied to the palm.

Some ointments provide pain relief, reduced muscular spasms, and increased mobility of affected arthritic joints through an anti-irritant effect. Ordinary cream only effectively soothes pain while the inflammation is still present. DMSO doesn't always operate in this manner. With DMSO, however, the skin's reaction, including irritations and inflammation, vanishes while the beneficial effects last for several hours.

An intriguing claim is that using DMSO on one problematic joint or area frequently results in pain relief in any other region. The effects of DMSO are widespread. It calms the central nervous system's terror response, and since it enters the bloodstream through the skin, it naturally reaches every part of the body.

In many regions of the world, DMSO is recommended as a treatment. For instance, DMSO became a legally prescribed drug for both humans and animals in the United States in 1978 and 1970, respectively.

In Canada, DMSO is used to treat scleroderma; in the UK and Ireland, it is used to treat shingles; in Germany and Austria, it is used to treat bursitis, tendinitis, and arthritis; in Switzerland, it is used to treat many disabilities while in Russia, it is used to treat a wide range of medical conditions.

Some persons with fair complexions, such as those with pink or blond hair and blue eyes, are more sensitive to DMSO. As such, it must be used on a 50% proportion or less for topical, oral, or intravenous application, particularly to the face and neck.

<h2 style="text-align:center"><u>CHAPTER EIGHT.</u></h2>

<h2 style="text-align:center"><u>DMSO THERAPY FOR INJURIES TO THE SPINAL CORD & STROKE.</u></h2>

With the use of standard techniques, severe recurrent accidents, especially those involving the spinal cord, are frequently difficult to handle. It is frequently impossible to determine how much if any, damage is done to the spinal cord as a result of vehicle accidents, workplace accidents, diving accidents, sports accidents, or other trauma until it is too late.

Back and neck injuries frequently result in complex medical problems that go far beyond the possibility of immediate spinal cord damage.

Treatment Strategy.

* ♣ The only DMSO treatment for spinal cord damage is an intravenous slow drip. Following DMSO intravenous administration properly will increase the amount of blood floating around the injury area.

* ♣ DMSO can also be applied locally to the spinal region or taken orally when mixed with juice or water.

* ♣ It is advisable to begin DMSO treatment immediately following the accident because there is a likelihood of permanent damage if treatment is delayed.

All stroke victims should most likely be treated with DMSO as it has several properties that make it useful for treating any mind-related health issues. Stroke is the second most common cause of death from cardiovascular disease, causing at least 500,000 more deaths a year in the US.

This abnormal system has many different aspects, ranging from stress, oxygen loss, insufficient blood flow, and blood drift to enzyme release.

A crucial quality of DMSO is its ability to cross the blood-brain barrier. It is one of the few products that can bypass this safety barrier. The barrier between the mind and the blood in circulation is known as the blood-mind barrier. It protects the brain against toxins that are harmful to the tissue therein.

There is typically an accumulation of water inside the brain as a result of the stroke because the damage destroys some of the cells. Different brain cells are compressed by the fluid accumulation inside the skull, leading to the death of more cells. More fluid is removed from the brain thanks to DMSO, which also lowers blood pressure and lessens damage to the brain.

An important factor to take into account is the fact that using DMSO has no negative side effects.

A lot of stroke victims' lives could be saved each year with the proper application of DMSO. Delaying treatment may result in death or permanent brain damage.

Even with a mild stroke, immediate treatment is advised. Instant DMSO treatment will reduce the risk of permanent damage in the event of a mild stroke. If the stroke is severe, immediate treatment with DMSO can frequently save a person's life or prevent permanent disability.

Treatment Strategy.

* Apply DMSO solution topically to the stroke victim's head within a few minutes of the attack. Try this for three to four months, every day. The DMSO treatment will cause the patient to begin to improve health-wise.

* In addition to the topical treatment, the patient must consume one teaspoon of DMSO daily for a period of six months to a year in a small glass of water.

* DMSO can also be given intramuscularly in addition to topical application.

CHAPTER NINE.

THERAPEUTICAL DMSO FOR BRAIN DAMAGE.

It may be very difficult to treat severe mental injuries with conventional techniques, including those brought on by falls, trauma, commercial accidents, and other accidents. Numerous problems are brought on by these mishaps, including:

- ☐ Nerve damage,
- ☐ The uncoordinated radical formation,
- ☐ Edema,
- ☐ Diminished blood gliding, and
- ☐ Oxygen loss.

DMSO is the simplest agent for treating severe brain injuries due to its unique properties.

Treatment Strategy.

Following the accident, DMSO treatment must begin. However, it is untrue that treatment must begin within 4 hours of an injury, contrary to claims made in some studies and books.

There is no particular amount of time. Generally speaking, the positive results are felt as soon as the damage has only begun to occur.

In this situation, sooner is better, and later is better than never.

When there is a long delay, there is typically permanent harm.

Brain tissue is incredibly delicate and may quickly deteriorate if it receives little oxygen. If treatment is postponed, a patient may lose all of their mental capacity or even pass away.

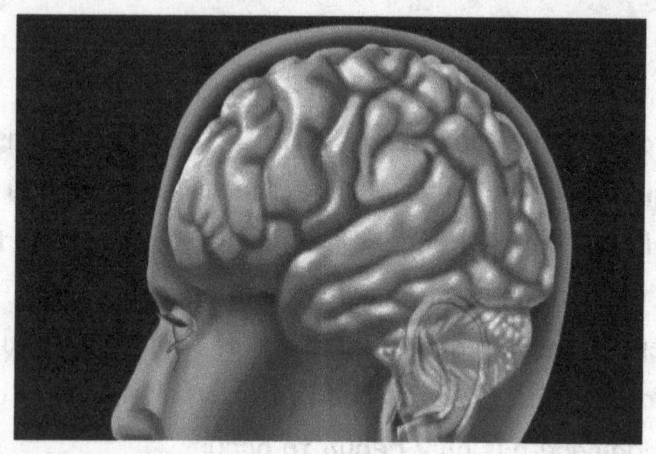

☐ The most popular DMSO treatment for severe brain injuries is the intravenous slow drip method. Up to 5grams per kilogram of body weight were given for 24 hours without any negative side effects. After the first 24 hours, reduce the dosage to 2 or 3 grams per kilogram of body weight per day.

☐ The principal portion of the DMSO dosage is typically given more quickly during the first hour of treatment on the first day of treatment.

DMSO TREATMENT FOR BRAIN-DAMAGED CHILDREN.

DMSO has proven to be helpful in cases of Down syndrome and intellectual disability. It penetrates the blood-brain barrier, which is a major obstacle to brain treatment and carries tablets through it. Additionally, some types of psychosis have been treated with it.

Oral DMSO is administered to mentally ill children at a 50% concentration. It is primarily helpful for babies with disabilities who receive 1/2gram per kg orally. The mother and father of the child will observe some degree of efficacy.

CHAPTER TEN.

DMSO THERAPY FOR MENTAL ILLNESS.

For over forty years, DMSO has been used to deal with sufferers with extreme psychiatric troubles consisting of:

* Schizophrenia,

- ♣   Alcoholic psychoses,
- ♣   Obsessive-compulsive neurosis,
- ♣   Excessive tension, and different intellectual troubles.

According to a DMSO study related to forty-two Peruvian sufferers. This observation covered 25 sufferers with schizophrenia, four with manic depressive psychotics, four with alcoholic psychotics, four with compulsive-obsessive neurotics, and five sufferers with excessive tension states.

A group of sixteen sufferers with comparable issues turned into shape haven used DMSO therapy. DMSO has been proven to soundly lessen the signs and symptoms of intellectual sufferers stricken by an extensive variety of issues. It's a product that must be utilized in all intellectual fitness facilities. Too many mentally challenged persons are admitted to psychiatric hospitals without a practical prospect of recovery.

With the right use of DMSO, lots of those sufferers may be helped to live efficient lifestyles out of the doors of the intellectual institution. There isn't any danger due to the fact there aren't any deadly or dangerous possible outcomes. To discover what works fine, extraordinary dosages and mixtures with diverse tablets and nutrients might be tried.

Treatment Strategy.

Before commencing any DMSO remedy, the sufferers ought to be taken off all preceding medicines for a minimum of one week.

* Oral administration: DMSO amino acid remedy may be administered orally in doses of 3 pills consistently on daily basis for six months.

* DMSO may be injected intravenously in 5% concentration doses of 3 ampoules weekly for about 15 days.

* The intravenous application can be repeated using the same method for 6 months.

* Giving a 5ml intramuscular injection of either 50% or 80% concentrations of DMSO solution twice or thrice daily.

* For highly troubled patients, you can administer about 5 injections daily.
* Patients with slight signs and symptoms can begin with 1 or 2 vials of 50% concentration of DMSO solution.
* As the signs enhance, all patients may be placed on an equal 50% concentration of DMSO solution doses.

CHAPTER ELEVEN.

SCIATICA AND LUMBA-DISC PROBLEM HEALING WITH DMSO THERAPY.

In instances of aching backs, particularly those involving disc illnesses that bring about excruciating spinal aches and often require surgery, research has shown that applying a DMSO solution can help reduce remedy time and strategies to a large extent.

Regular injection of at least 20ml-50ml of 20% DMSO applied alongside an anesthetic xylocaine to the injury spot, will help a great deal compared to other remedies. You can as well use the Intravenous method every 2-3 days.

BURNS, SCARS, AND KELOID TREATMENT WITH DMSO THERAPY.

The elevated nodular, lobulated linear mass of scar tissue in keloids is flattened by DMSO when applied topically and frequently, and this further removes any discolorations. Even though it won't eliminate the parallel bands of heavily collagenous fabric, it will help. It can also help to minimize scarring from persistent pimples where fibrous papules have developed on the hair follicle's surface, typically around the hairline at the lower back of the neck.

In a study done on ten patients with keloids, using an 80% concentration of DMSO solution repeatedly throughout the day caused the collagen surrounding the fibrous bundles to relax. DMSO can help prevent adhesions/scars brought on by prior surgery. This could be accomplished by surgically injecting a diluted DMSO solution into the stomach cavity.

Burns are injuries to the tissue caused by chemicals, electrical impact, radiation, or heat. *There are many degrees of burns; first-degree burns, second-degree burns that can be treated from the comfort of the home, and third-degree burns that frequently require specialized medical care.*

Treatment Strategy.

- Apply a 50% concentration of DMSO lotion mixed with a 50% concentration of Aloe-vera immediately after the burn injury occurred.

- After one hour, apply the same content. Do this every 3 hours for 2 days. This will help heal the burn victim.

Using DMSO lotion mixed with aloe vera, helps you avoid blister formation on the burnt area. Sunburns can be treated with DMSO as well. The majority of physicians who use DMSO to treat serious burns have concluded that creams with DMSO and aloe vera in their content often give a more positive recovery result. The mixture helps to lessen, dissolve, or even prevent scar tissue development; a major after-effect of burn injuries.

CHAPTER TWELVE.

FUNGI INFECTION TREATMENT WITH DMSO.

In the treatment of fungal infections and other skin-related ailments, DMSO can be quite effective. It has been used as an effective remedy for several skin ailments, jungle rot, zits/acne as well as athlete's foot.

Jungle rot is a foot contamination that mostly occurs in hot, humid climates season. It was discovered during World War II when a veteran was infected with it during service in the South Pacific.

According to him, he has spent so much of his personal and government resources that were made available for him, in a bid to get a cure for this ailment which proves abortive until he used a DMSO skin lotion mixed with aloe vera and then came a great relief for him. Although the lotion did not cure the ailment totally, it provided a more positive result and relief compared to other medications that were used.

This therapy was later used by a Los Angeles-based doctor for the Veterans Administration to treat several veterans which yielded positive results. Although subsequent infection occurred because the fungi weren't eliminated.

An athlete's foot is another fungal infection that responds properly to DMSO treatment. It is a common chronic ailment that gets worse throughout the summer, particularly when enclosed foot wares are frequently worn thereby preventing the escape of heat and moisture.

Treatment Strategy.

- Topically apply a 50% to 90% concentration of DMSO lotion to the affected area. In addition to DMSO, aloe vera and capsicum pepper can be used once in a while.
- To treat the fungus under the fingernails and toenails, topically apply DMSO to the nail and the arms or feet around the contaminated area.
- Apply the treatment twice daily till the fungi clear up.

CANCER THERAPY USING DMSO.

DMSO solution has been used over the years to treat cancer ailment with positive relief outcome and it happens to be one of the most important products for treating cancer that is readily available in the market today with numerous properties that makes it potent. It is an effective detoxifier and free radical scavenger.

It can interact with several other medications while also bypassing body tissue and individual cells inside the body. While DMSO is anti-cancer on its own, it is significantly more effective when combined with other possible anti-cancer medicines.

Treatment Strategy.

* To prevent some side effects of cancer treatment, 70% to 90% concentration of DMSO should be applied 3-8hours per day for 10 to 14 days with proper medical guidance.

* Add a small dosage of cyclophosphamide and DMSO in some water and administer about 4mg per kg of the body weight to the patient daily or regularly till a maximum of 4gm has been administered. Always watch out for any negative side effects while treatment is on.

- ♣ Repeat another cycle of treatment until a 3-4grms has been administered haven stopped the injection for 12-15 days.

Note: Repetition of treatment depends solely on the absence or reduction of the ailment or the general health condition of the patient.

Patients with diabetic ailments who have in time past used DMSO solution as a treatment remedy reported positive outcomes. Although this doesn't stop the use of insulin though some patients with this condition were able to require less insulin through the regular usage of DMSO. *However, it is inadvisable to discontinue the use of insulin without speaking to your physician.* The importance of using DMSO as a treatment measure for diabetics stems from its ability to reduce diabetic neuropathy, a loss in classic sensory nerve features often found in older diabetic patients.

One out of every four young people with diabetes who use topical DMSO may experience a decrease in the need for insulin. This enhances blood delivery via dilation of the tiny blood arteries, mostly inside the lower limbs. The medication should be part of the pre-surgical preparations when the healthcare professional wants to increase the blood supply to a portion of the diabetic patient's body.

Treatment Strategy.

- Massage the DMSO lotion to the feet and legs twice per day.
- Every night after dinner, put a teaspoon of DMSO solution into a juice cup and consume it.
- Regularly work out, and stick to your weight-loss plan.

Within a few weeks, tremendous changes will be seen.

HEADACHE TREATMENT WITH DMSO.

Complications can affect people at any point in their life. In actuality, at least half of the population experiences headaches once a month. Muscle spasms in the neck and changes in the blood arteries leading to the head are the main causes of headaches.

The body's reaction to emotional stress and how it affects it are frequently the underlying causes. Aspirin is the first line of treatment for headache patients. The resultant effect may differ, but there's usually minimal pain relief.

DMSO has been used to address headache issues for several years. In comparison to many conventional painkillers, the effects are frequently of excellent quality with fewer side effects.

Completely developed migraine problems don't often respond well to treatment. However, it has been found that DMSO can turn the situation around if a migraine headache is treated at an early stage. This has happened to many people with the condition. Treatment must begin as soon as the ache is noticed.

<u>**Treatment Strategy.**</u>

Common DMSO treatment patterns for headaches include;

* Massaging DMSO solution on the head, neck region, or both aside from the face.

* One teaspoon of DMSO can be added to 4 ounces of water and consumed daily or administered intravenously (via injection) or by having the patient drink it in juice or water.

* Continue with this treatment pattern for a maximum of 6 months till the pain fades off completely.

<u>CHAPTER THIRTEEN.</u>

<u>DMSO THERAPY FOR HERPES, SHINGLES, CATARACT AND EYE RELATED PROBLEMS.</u>

Herpes virus and other viral infections can be successfully treated with DMSO or by combining it with other anti-inflammatory and anti-viral drugs. Shingles, commonly known as herpes zoster, can be extremely harmful in most cases and they are caused by a virus that leads to chickenpox in the victim. Before a patient's full recovery from this disease, it often lasts for weeks and can also result in blindness to the patients when the disease spreads to the facial region.

Postherpetic neuralgia is a disorder that can develop after the shingles lesions have healed. The agony from this can be unbearably bad and last for years. Postherpetic neuralgia pain can be reduced but not completely eradicated by DMSO and other drugs. Preventing post-herpetic neuralgia is one of the key components of shingles treatment. The quickest possible shingles treatment is the greatest approach to preventing neuralgia development.

In a study carried out on patients with persistent skin ulcers in Chile, major factors that contributed to their skin ulcers were burns, infected wounds, and diabetic sores. Most of the burns had become infected. Many of the sores have been there for some time with adequate medication to heal them up previously until DMSO was used alongside other antibiotics and anti-inflammatory medications that were sprayed on the wounds.

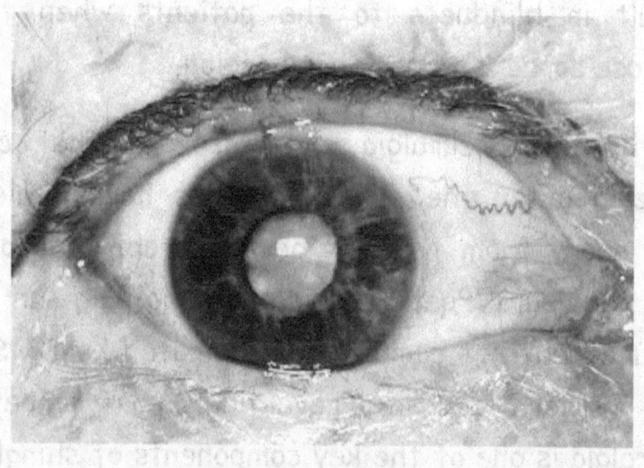

Treatment Strategy.

☐ Spray the affected area with a mixture of DMSO, antibiotics, and an anti-inflammatory medication 3 times weekly.

☐ When this treatment is being applied, there may be some pain, but it only lasts for a while although most patients experience relief right away.

- Apply a lotion mixed with DMSO, aloe vera, and eucalyptus oil on both legs twice daily for a month if you have severe varicose ulcers on both legs.

- For treating animals, apply the lotion on the animal's skin and the affected area.

TREATING CATARACTS AND OTHER EYE PROBLEMS.

The use of DMSO to treat cataracts and other eye issues such as traumatic uveitis (an inflammation of the pigmented part of the eye), macular edema, and macular degeneration (deterioration of the macula-lutea, a portion of the retina), has been quite successful throughout the years.

In ophthalmology, DMSO has been injected into the intraocular region of the eye to treat corneal edema successfully. The retina is a thin layer that covers roughly two-thirds of the inner surface of the eyeball and a portion of the eye that is sensitive to light. DMSO is a useful remedy for retinal diseases such as eye deterioration, degeneration, dystrophy, and bio-trophy, all of which are non-inflammatory types of retinal abnormalities.

DMSO healing capacity for retina diseases was discovered when some patients with retinitis pigmentosa; a retinal disease, who were receiving DMSO treatment for some musculoskeletal disorders, noticed that their vision had improved while on the drug.

Investigation about this medication began properly when some researchers reported that a patient with retinitis pigmentosa experienced a very stunning improvement in vision following the application of DMSO in a Los Angeles study on the prevention of blindness.

<u>**Treatment Strategy.**</u>

- Apply one drop of DMSO solution of 40% concentration, once daily, using an eyedropper (this can be used for any eye-related ailments).

- There might be some stinging sensation after applying the solution, but it will fade off after some time, and a great relief afterward.

- For cataract issues, apply a drop of DMSO directly to the affected eye.

- For cases of cataract and glaucoma, mix about 25mg of DMSO with 2 drops of SOD (Super-Oxide Dismutase) and apply one drop of the mixture to the affected eye.

CHAPTER FOURTEEN.

DMSO REMEDY FOR HAIR, SCALP PROBLEMS, AND PAINS.

The potential of DMSO to dramatically lessen pain is one of its most important benefits. In cases where the pain is a major problem, this chapter of the book is the answer.

Pain is the body's electrochemical alarm indicator that something is wrong. It notifies the body of the presence of anything with the potential to cause damage or harm to tissues in the body. DMSO typically has a substantial analgesic effect. Nevertheless, it is very important to identify the main cause of the pain.

The use of DMSO is not meant to replace medical care. Even if the source of a patient's continuous discomfort cannot be determined, there is still a problem. DMSO is not the appropriate treatment for an appendicitis patient. It is important to get medical help as soon as possible. In an emergency, surgery can be the best option to save the patient's life. The full potential of DMSO may be utilized once the cause of the discomfort has been identified.

<u>Treatment Strategy.</u>

- Topically apply a 90% concentration of DMSO lotion 2 times daily on the patient's entire back for a minimum of 6 months or even more, depending on how much relief you feel while the treatment is on.

While following through with this treatment plan, always visit your therapist to know the level of progress obtained.

<u>TREATMENT WITH DMSO FOR HAIR AND SCALP PROBLEMS.</u>

DMSO has been in use for over 4 decades to promote hair growth. Patients with lost hairlines often experience positive outcomes. When hair grows, new hair first appears in the areas where the most hair has been lost. There was rapid hair growth among cancer patients who lost their hair due to chemotherapy impact when DMSO lotion was applied to their head to the amazement of the oncologist.

He further allowed them to continue using the DMSO drug with the confidence that it wouldn't cause any harm to them and the patients were also eager to have their hair grow back. The same thing applies to animals fed with DMSO.

This happens because DMSO has vasodilator potency that helps dilate those tiny capillaries inside the scalp. This enhances the increase in blood flow to the hair roots. The hair follicles are subsequently given nutrients, allowing hair to grow again. With typical male pattern baldness, hair growth is usually slow, but many patients have reported positive results. After using DMSO on the head, there has been no contamination for six months, and the scalp has improved.

DMSO THERAPY WITH PREGNANCY.

Although there haven't been any reliable studies on DMSO used for expectant mothers however if taken it is necessary, to ensure that its benefits outweigh the risks to the unborn child.

CHAPTER FIFTEEN.

HEARING AND EAR IMPAIRMENT TREATMENT WITH DMSO.

A great number of persons out there who experiences one ear issue or the other include children and adults. In a normal situation, puncturing the eardrum to discharge pus and ease its tension is a common solution to this situation but it always comes with excruciating pain.

However, the eardrum can often be perforated without the usual intense pain when DMSO is combined with an anesthetic. In other cases, DMSO plus an antibiotic can be used to treat patients with middle or internal ear infections without puncturing the eardrum.

Treatment Strategy.

* Pour a 50% concentration of DMSO solution into an eyedropper and put 2 drops of the solution inside each ear.
* Topically rub a 90% concentration of DMSO solution around the head and neck region close to the ears. Repeat this process twice daily until great relief is obtained.

<u>**TINNITUS TREATMENT USING DMSO THERAPY.**</u>

Tinnitus is one major reason why people visit ear, nose, and throat specialists. It is a condition whereby a patient complains of numerous ear disturbances. The most common sounds include; hissing, buzzing, or ringing noises as well as other varied sounds. The issue may be persistent or irregular, often leading to a partial loss of hearing in the victim. The affected person's physical and mental health may suffer greatly if the noise becomes regular and tough.

There was not much that could be done to lessen tinnitus symptoms before the use of DMSO. Occasionally, surgical intervention was attempted. In another instance, the doctors thought the problem was likely caused by contamination and tried several antibiotics without results.

<u>**Treatment Strategy.**</u>

* Drop some amount of DMSO solution alongside an anti-inflammatory and

vasodilator medicine inside the ear canal every 4-days for one month

♣ Take a daily dosage of DMSO intramuscular injection.

<u>CHAPTER SIXTEEN</u>

<u>SPORTS INJURY AND INTERSTITIAL CYSTITIS HEALING POTENTIAL OF DMSO.</u>

Applying DMSO treatment to sport-related injuries such as; dislocations, strains, tennis elbow, severe cuts, and several other injuries provides great relief. In cases of acute trauma, pain is rapidly eased, swelling reduced, and functions returned.

TRAUMA HEALING IN SPORTS.

DMSO has more benefits than just acting as an anti-inflammatory agent and painkiller. Studies revealed that it can lessen swellings in the victim.

70-80 percent of those who utilize this drug for soccer injuries often obtain excellent recovery results. The injured players immediately feel less pain; reducing swelling and further hastening their recovery.

The athletes detected these benefits by comparing their most recent injuries, for which they received DMSO, to earlier injuries of a similar kind.

A 70% concentration of DMSO is an excellent medication that appears to significantly reduce the amount of time needed for recovery after sports-related injuries to joints or other soft tissues of the body. It contributes positively to those working in commercial medicine and sports medicine because returning people to their regular activities as soon as feasible is one of their top priorities.

The ability to recover injured persons more quickly than usual is the main benefit of using DMSO therapy. This will help save hundreds of persons with occupational injuries and bring them back to work earlier than normal.

INTERSTITIAL CYSTITIS HEALING WITH DMSO.

Interstitial cystitis is an inflammation of the interior lining of the bladder. In 1978, the FDA approved the use of DMSO particularly as a treatment for interstitial cystitis. Before this period, there was no sure treatment for interstitial cystitis.

Its symptoms resemble that of cystitis; a common bacterial infection that can be properly treated with antibiotic medication. However, interstitial cystitis isn't usually caused by bacteria hence, it does not respond to antibiotic treatment. The most common and widely applied treatment for this condition is DMSO. Extreme bladder symptoms such as scarring, bleeding, and decreased bladder capacity can be caused by interstitial cystitis.

The pain oftentimes can be intense, particularly when the bladder gets filled to the bream and thereafter, reduces when urine is passed out. Some patients usually feel the urge to urinate up to fifty times daily day and night to get relief.

The directive for the usage of DMSO when it was initially approved for use in the treatment of interstitial cystitis was by using a syringe/tube to immediately inject the drug into the patient's bladder a few times per week. However, some patients complain of severe pain using this method.

Hence, it could no longer be used further and the oral method was adopted i.e. oral take DMSO solution with a teaspoon of juice or water. Because it is far less unpleasant for the patient, many doctors agree that taking DMSO orally is the best way to treat interstitial cystitis.

Treatment Strategy.

* Mix DMSO in cranberry juice and take a teaspoon orally 1-2 times daily.

* Both the intravenous and oral treatment methods can also be used; begin treatment with the bladder instillation and follow up with the oral treatment after-was.

CHAPTER SEVENTEEN.

THERAPEUTICAL DMSO FOR ARTHRITIS AND SHINGLES.

DMSO is far from being a useless substance. It appears to function as a local analgesic and may therefore be helpful in other painful circumstances. Although no scientific proof has been documented as to whether it lessens inflammation and swelling, which are essential in rheumatoid arthritis, or that it changes the fundamental development of whatever connective tissue illness.

This resulted in the restriction of DMSO usage for patients with rheumatoid arthritis and other types of arthritis disorders by the Arthritis Foundation stating that the patients need more than a pain relief medication; there's a need for the irritation to be subdued which aspirin application in its right dosage can help achieve that compared to DMSO.

Treatment Strategy.

* In Osteoarthritis: Topically apply a 25% concentration of DMSO gel three times per day, or

♣ Practice the 45.5% concentration of the DMSO application method 4 times daily.

TREATMENT FOR DIGESTIVE ISSUES.

Different types of digestive illnesses can be difficult to identify and even more difficult to treat.

A simple method of treating this ailment using DMSO solution is to take half a teaspoon of DMSO solution mixed with 1 ounce of Aloe-vera and diluted with 2 ounces of water every morning after breakfast for 2 weeks (14 days).

SHINGLES THERAPY USING DMSO.

Shingle is a viral infection known as subsoil which results in a painful rash. This illness can manifest itself on the body in the form of a fester anywhere.

Typically, only a small section of one side of the body is affected by shingles symptoms. The symptoms include;

- ♣ Feeling pain,
- ♣ Burning,
- ♣ Touch sensitivity,
- ♣ Formation of a red rash several days after the pain has passed,
- ♣ Itchiness from liquid blisters that eventually break apart.

One of DMSO's best-known properties is its quick skin absorption capacity. DMSO can be utilized to enhance the pain-relieving components of specific elements because it helps boosts their potency and efficiency. However, we must apply caution when combining components with DMSO to observe how it impacts you since side effects can also be improved.

<u>**Treatment Strategy.**</u>

- ☐ The drug can be used in the following dosages.
- ☐ Combine a 5% to 40% solution of idoxuridine with DMSO and topically apply it on the afflicted area within 48 hours of the rash appearing. Repeat this method every 4 hours for 4 days respectively.

When using an already-made cream, ensure you follow the instructions and usage directives as written in the cream manual. Always start with a lower dosage and then gradually increase the dosage while keeping your body's response to the medicine (DMSO) in check.

CHAPTER EIGHTEEN.

DMSO REMEDY FOR LEG, FOOT AND SLUDGE INJURIES.

☐ Bunions In The Big Toe.

A bunion (hallux valgus) is simply a bony bump that forms at the base of the big toe joint as a result of the diversion of two connected bones, most frequently at the first metatarsal joint. It is an inflammation of the bursa-sac *(a sac that contains fluid like an egg white)*; a lubricant between the skin and the bone. The sac becomes swollen from continuous irritation from an external force, like an ill-fitted further resulting in an acute and painful condition.

Its symptoms include;

- ☐ Bone deformity,
- ☐ Pain and
- ☐ Bone stiffness.

A bunion is basically of two types;

- ☐ Severe Bunion.
- ☐ Chronic Bunion.

The acute bunion is usually unanticipated and painful and if not properly treated, it can resort to a chronic bunion also known as the hallux valgus or habitual bunion. Unlike the acute bunion, the chronic bunion is a simple deformity of the big toe which is often painless. However, it can be painful in most cases.

It widens the foot, which throws one off balance and makes standing and walking quite difficult. As a result of this disorder, foot arthritis may appear early in childhood. Osteoarthritis develops as a result of persistently ignoring the big toe bunion. Wearing larger shoes is the only way to accommodate the deformity caused by calcification at stress sites and common enlargement. With DMSO therapy, the acute stage of a bunion can be improved upon.

Treatment Strategy.

- ☐ Get a plastic cover to fit under the foot.
- ☐ Apply DMSO solution at the base of the affected foot and wrap the foot with the plastic cover.
- ☐ Ensure it is properly secured with protective padding and leave it for 3 days.

DMSO REMEDY FOR HARD AND SOFT SLUDGE.

Soft sludge grows between the toes and on the coverings of the toes, while hard sludge is excessive skin growth. Both types can be easily differentiated from their surrounding soft tissue. Pain is one major symptom of this ailment. About

40 percent of patients who visits the podiatrist do so mainly for hard and soft sludge issues of which female takes the larger amount of those patients.

Disunion and pressure brought on by an elevated undermining bone result in the formation of sludge. Uncomfortable shoes hurt the skin on the outside while the sharp edge of the toe bone irritates the skin from the inside. In the end, the epidermis decomposes, and the sludge develops gradually as the pains and aches get tensed.

<u>Treatment Strategy.</u>

- ☐ Sludge victims may find temporary or long-term relief from their symptoms using the DMSO solution. Although it doesn't give a permanent cure.
- ☐ Shave off the uncomfortable wanton on the skin and topically apply DMSO solution on the shaved area.

CHAPTER NINETEEN

DMSO REMEDY FOR FOOT-TOENAILS.

Thick, ugly, and misshaped toenails might be signs of a systemic condition or a persistent injury in older persons, just like running in improperly fitted handled shoes. As a result of injury, toenails are constantly discolored, stretched, and thickened.

Toenails that have become too long are often referred to as club nails. They can coil beneath the toes, strong and looking like a ram horn. To avoid building a dwelling home for girdling parasitic fungus, it is best to maintain a short toenail as possible.

<u>Treatment Strategy.</u>

☐ Mix 90% concentration of DMSO solution with warm castor oil or warm olive oil and topically apply to the affected nail. It will help soften the nails.

☐ Reapply the mixture again after the first treatment to give a lasting feeling of comfort and restore squeezed tissues to normalcy.

Simple steps in preventing club nails disease:

- Keep your toenails short by trimming regularly.
- Use toenail clippers for trimming
- Apply one drop of DMSO solution to the edge of the nails after cutting.

DMSO REMEDY FOR FUNGI-INFECTED TOENAILS.

Toenail fungi infections are among the most typical nail issues. This kind of nail issue affects one out of every four adults above age thirty who visit the podiatrist. It results from parasitic infections like yeast, mold, or fungi which further grow as ringworm. These parasites are often harbored in clothing items like shoes; the shoe is one material that is hardly cleaned inside.

Fungi-infected toenails look;

- Dry.
- Scaly.
- Dull.
- Elevated from the nail base,
- Yellowish-brown.

Because the infection extends back toward the nail root as it advances, the entire nail or only a portion of it may be impacted.

Treatment Strategy.

* Orally take antibiotic griseofulvin.
* Ironize the affected nail with copper sulfate.

- ♣ Apply fungicide to the affected area; either in liquid or ointment form.
- ♣ Depending on its severity, the affected nail can be removed permanently or temporarily. If removed temporarily, direct the treatment to the nail base and the growth center where a new nail can grow without fungi infection.
- ♣ Combine 30% concentration of DMSO and 2 small sizes of 250mg griseofulvin tablets to create a paste and massage it on the nail surrounding once the nail base has healed up. Use a band to hold the mixture (paste) in place. New uninfected toenails should grow out from under the skin for several months following this procedure.
- ♣ Continually apply the paste mixture to the nail base daily for 6 months till the new toenail develops completely.
- ♣ The healed nail base can also be treated with DMSO combined with other liquid fungicides.

CHAPTER TWENTY.

DMSO TREATMENT FOR ATHLETIC FOOT DISEASE.

This is a medical condition also known as "tinea pedis". Tinea means "fungus" while pedis means "foot". Athletic foot disease simply describes a set of symptoms rather than the underlying reason.

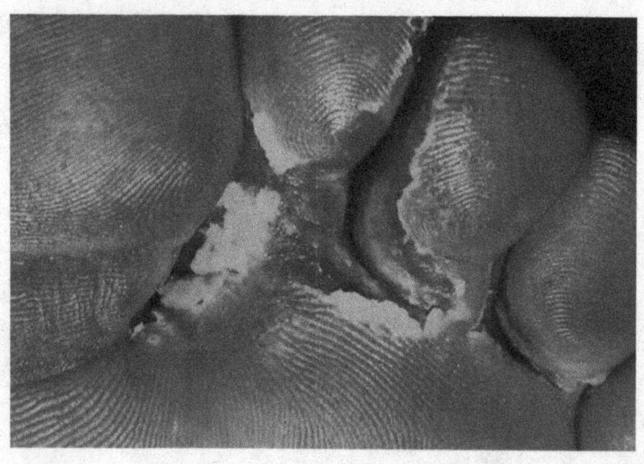

Tinea does not cause foot disease on its own, it only strives for a favorable dwelling environment as a parasite and the foot that is always in an enclosed shoe happens to be that favorable environment to dwell in. It is mostly found on the feet of men compared to women whose shoes are usually more open than men's.

<u>Signs:</u>

- Scaling around the toes and edges of the heels,

- Folded skin.

- Wrinkle and shell

- Clustered tiny blisters that rupture with time and reveal shiny red circular areas under the feed.

For every four out of five infected individuals, the symptoms recur consistently from one warm season to the next in 80% of cases. Antifungal treatments administered under the feet with DMSO as the carrier agent happens to be a superb type of treatment for this disease. DMSO as the carrier agent helps kill any fungus on the skin's surface or inside the skin by penetrating the upper skin layers and delivering the antifungal agent deeply into the tissues. Similarly, DMSO, a fungistatic agent, inhibits athlete's foot symptoms by stifling the development of the troublesome parasite.

Treatment Strategy.

* Apply the appropriate athlete's foot lotion to dress the affected skin,
* Open up the skin,
* Apply an ointment on the scaly area, thick skin, and the blisters,

* Mix DMSO in a cream, gel, or liquid and apply it to the infected area.

* Apply 70% concentration of DMSO solution topically to enhance the penetration power of the antifungal agent. Following these procedures will help elevate the disease greatly.

DMSO TREATMENT FOR FOOT ODOR.

One of the most annoying problems is foot odor, even though it is not harmful or communicable. It is referred to as bromidrosis in science. It is mainly caused by physiological issues which disrupt the neurological functioning system. It brings humiliation to its victims thereby inhibiting their social life. Uncleanliness does not affect foot odor, but good foot hygiene can help lessen the foul smell.

A foot odor victim needs more than just washing the feet to eliminate the foul smell.

Symptoms of Foot Odor;

- Offensive smell.

- Stuffy skin between toes.

- Foot flesh tenderness.

- Tiny blisters on feet balls.

__Treatment Strategy.__

Foot odor does not heal quickly after treatment. But there are ways to lessen the issue and eliminate it in most cases.

* ♣ Apply 50% concentration of DMSO topically to the base of the feet; it may seem as though you are merely substituting one unpleasant smell (garlic-like odor from the DMSO solution) with another (smell from the feet) but the odor from DMSO will fade off in few days leaving the feet odor free.

* ♣ The best solution to foot odor is to eliminate sugar from your diet and supplement with B complex vitamins and zinc to receive immediate relief.

CHAPTER TWENTY-ONE.

CHAPTER TWENTY-ONE.

DMSO TREATMENT FOR PAIN AND ANKLE SPRAIN.

A common ailment brought on by a rough wringing of the foot is a sprained ankle. You can unintentionally sprain your ankle while strolling down the street, by jumping from any height or treading on a rough surface depending on how active you are.

Sprain generally occurs when the foot is out of balance leading to a twist in the foot. After a sprain, the signs and symptoms of an injury start to show. Any weight that is immediately applied to the hurt foot may cause pain. If the sprain is slight, the ankle becomes sensitive and uncomfortable.

However, if the sprain is severe, the ankle could become hot and blown. As the lump expands, palpitations accompany it. You can begin seeking urgent home care for a sprained ankle even before visiting the hospital.

<u>**Treatment Strategy.**</u>

* Have a sit and remove all weighty substances from the ankle.

* Apply 90% concentration of DMSO on the affected area. Although you could experience some burning or see some greenish discoloration, the pain of inflammation will eventually go away. Because symptoms don't often show up at once, it's not always feasible to pinpoint how severe the injury is; so be careful not to put much weight on the injured ankle.

* Although the sprain might be for a moment, particularly with the immediate application of DMSO therapy, utilizing the ankle could

98

make the situation worse. Therefore, do not take the chance.

- ♣ The DMSO will either lessen the swelling or prevent it from developing at all.

- ♣ After applying DMSO, properly support the sprained ankle by wrapping the band/gauze across the spot with DMSO solution using a napkin or apron.

  NOTE... Treating the pain isn't the same as repairing a sprain; assistance is required to keep the torn ligaments stocked to the leg bone and further prevent excessive movement.

Follow this treatment procedure every 4 days;

- Change the napkin/apron used in wrapping the ankle,
- Clean the skin surface,
- Reapply DMSO and wrap with a fresh napkin/apron.

Continue this treatment until you feel no pain from direct pressure impact.

<u>DMSO AS A BACK PAIN TREATMENT.</u>

Pains in the back region have a wide variety of causes. Among the most frequent are strains, injuries, age factors, and recurring illnesses like osteoporosis or arthritis. Two additional significant but generally disregarded reasons for backaches are over-acidity in the body, wrong sitting posture, and an improper resting position. Research has shown that most cases of back pain can be treated with antibiotics.

<u>Treatment Strategy.</u>

There are a lot of natural methods that can be used to treat back pain without having to go for antibiotics, like; reducing acidity levels and maintaining a good sleeping/sitting posture. While DMSO on the other hand can help reduce swelling, inflammation, and pains as well as speed up the healing process.

* Get a 99.9% concentration of pure liquid DMSO and mix it with distilled (purified) water.

- ♣ For a perfect solution: mix a 70% DMSO concentration and 30% purified water or mix a 90% DMSO concentration with 10% purified water.

- ♣ Apply this mixture topically by dabbing it with a cotton pad on the skin. For acute injuries, follow this procedure for 5 days every 2 hours between 6-8 hours following the injury.

- ♣ For quick absorption of the solution to the skin, rub a 50% concentration of DMSO in a volume of 1/3 teaspoon on the affected area rather than dabbing.

- ♣ In cases of nerve pain, topically apply 50% DMSO solution 4 times daily for about 3 weeks.

CHAPTER TWENTY-TWO.
RESPIRATORY, HEAD, AND SPINAL CORD INJURIES TREATMENT WITH DMSO.

Incisions or cuts across the spinal cord are usually very dangerous injuries that will unavoidably render the victim permanently disabled. All sensory and autonomic system functions below the damaged site are lost as a result of an acute transverse cord lesion, which also causes instantaneous limp palsy.

For several hours or days, limp palsy gradually changes into discontinuous paraplegia as a result of a magnified stretch kickback, robotic leaps, or branch spasms occur. Later, extensor, flexor, or muscular spasms develop, and deep tendon revulsions and autonomic revulsions gradually return if the spinal cord in the lumbosacral area isn't disassociated. Only partial motor and sensitive whim-whams loss may occur, depending on how severe the cord trauma is. The injured section of the spinal tract determines the degree of sensitivity loss; voluntary movement may return but it will be disorganized, resulting in the loss of certain sensational feelings such as vibration, pain, touches, or posture on the affected side. The indicators of recovery are there if there is any movement or sensation during the first week after the accident.

Any dysfunction that still exists six months later is likely to never end. Any injury above the fifth cervical chines is usually serious, and dangerous and may lead to death in most cases.

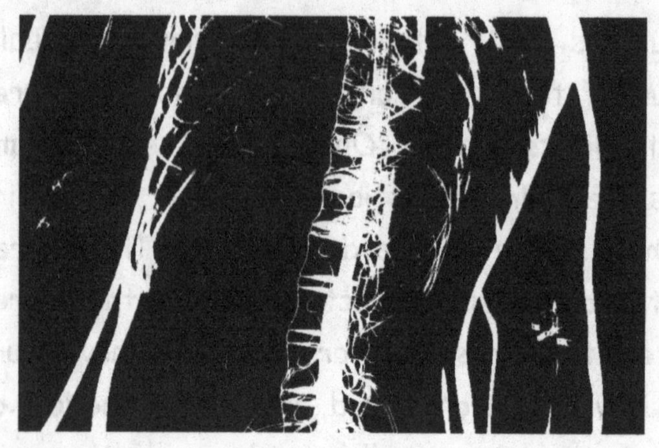

Intravenously apply DMSO solution within 90 minutes of the accident.

DMSO AS A TREATMENT FOR RESPIRATORY ISSUES.

Numerous people in the United States and other nations across the world are affected significantly by respiratory issues. These illnesses are particularly harmful to infants and the elderly. DMSO in combination with other medications like antibiotics and an anti-inflammatory medication has been proven effective in treating this health challenge to a very large extent.

Sixty infants with severe bronchiolitis participated in research to determine the effectiveness of adding DMSO to the conventional course of treatment. Two groups were formed from these infants. Thirty of the infants (control group) received therapy, oxygen, and antibiotics treatment in a brume tent while a DMSO aerosol spray, antibiotics, and an anti-inflammatory drug were given to the other group of 30 infants (DMSO Group). Treatment with DMSO resulted in quick healing. Eighty percent (80%) of the infants had improved greatly within 30 minutes of using DMSO. There was a reduction in coughing, the respiratory rate was reduced to about seventy-five percent (75%), and the breathing pattern was restored to normalcy.

There was a great benefit that was remitted because the DMSO group did not bear the cost of using the brume tent, unlike the control group. The DMSO spray used helped the respiratory process easier to cough up, which also decreased their thickness. Researchers, therefore, concluded that using a DMSO remedial spray to treat bronchiolitis is beneficial since it is easy to administer, has no harmful effects, and has positive clinical outcomes for acute respiratory obstructive processes.

A three-year-old boy who was severely ill with a high temperature, and cough was one of the kids who received treatment at the hospital. The decision was made to administer 1ml of DMSO spray to him via a tracheal cannula as his condition deteriorated further. He responded with fierce coughing and almost suffocating. His respiration steadily improved after some time and was later discharged from the hospital after some days having been declared fit medically.

The most prevalent chronic condition among children is asthma though it can affect people of different ages. Breathing might become so difficult during a severe asthmatic crisis that the patient may pass away from oxygen deprivation. The focus of conventional medical treatment for asthma has mostly been on relieving its symptoms. Anti-inflammatory drugs and cortisone are used to avert mucus building up, which can completely block inhalation in severe situations while inhalers help to open up the victim's airways. While these medications can save lives during an emergency if used frequently and for a long time, they may have unfavorable side effects.

Treatment Strategy.

Without the side effects related to cortisone and bronchodilators, DMSO is useful in treating asthma. This is consistently accomplished in a remarkably easy way, much like topical DMSO operation alone or in conjunction with other medications.

* Topically apply a mixture of DMSO lotion, an aloe vera gel, and eucalyptus oil on the nose region, chest, and forehead every night before going to bed.
* Avoid dehydration.

* Avoid alcoholic beverages and coffee drinks because they do not fall into the categories of liquids that help dehydrates the body.

CHAPTER TWENTY-THREE.

DMSO TREATMENT FOR THE TOOTH, INTRACRANIAL HYPERTENSION AND GUM PAINS.

Tooth and gum diseases (periodontal) are the leading cause of tooth loss in persons between their 40s and 50s. It is an inflammatory disorder in the gum-supporting tissues which progresses to gingivitis in its early stage of development. The disease affects the gums, supporting structures of the teeth as well as the periodontal membrane.

Plaque, which is a composite of thousands of living bacteria, forms as a result of bacteria feeding on food patches surrounding the gums. This results in gingival development (space between the tooth and the gum) thereby making the gums swell and start bleeding.

The bacteria feed on food patches that are left in the patient's mouth after eating to survive. It further expels waste, leaving feces and dirt on the teeth. This is what causes a person with a gum complaint to have an unpleasant mouth odor.

If the plaque is not properly treated, it spreads to the bone and membrane beneath the gum leading to severe damage to the tooth and the gum.

<u>**What Causes This?**</u>

The most frequent reasons for tooth and gum diseases include but are not limited to;

- Poor diet; excessive intake of processed sugar.
- Poor oral hygiene.

Therefore, regular brushing of the teeth using a 50% concentration of DMSO greatly slows the growth of germs. DMSO has been used successfully throughout history to treat gum and tooth issues.

* After brushing the teeth, apply a compress with DMSO of about 30% concentration for a minimum of 10 minutes every day for about 7-10 days.
* Topically rub DMSO solution on the outer surface of the gum (the cheek or jaw area).

TREATING INTRACRANIAL HYPERTENSION USING DMSO.

DMSO as a healing agent has been very effective in treating and reducing intracranial hypertension (high blood pressure in the skull) caused by head trauma as described by several neurological experts.

Six patients were used as an experiment to ascertain the potency of this drug; 2 of the 6 patients were given an intravenous injection of 10% concentration of DMSO while the other 4 patients received a 20% concentration titrate (determined by drops counting). Five of these cases included severe head injuries, and one involved a cortical venous thrombosis (a pregnancy-related blood clot in the cerebral cortex).

This delivery method improved ICP management, although, despite a high level of alertness, difficulties with fluid function and electrolytes recurred. DMSO's solvent properties and tendency to dissolve (lower concentration capacity) in the majority of conventional IV infusion systems over time also contributed to the mechanical challenges associated with its administration that were present in all six cases.

The mechanism of action in DMSO is quite unclear compared to barbiturates, it performs too swiftly to be used as a diuretic alone. The medication is highly difficult to administer, and eventually, difficulties with administration can cause its drawbacks to outweigh its inherent advantages. Therefore, the use of DMSO to treat intracranial hypertension should be postponed until more laboratory data are available and better delivery techniques are created, according to neurosurgeons.

Both oral and intravenous methods of DMSO administration have an impact on children's memory and brain development and the elaboration of their intellectual skills, preparing them for academic activities.

<u>**CHAPTER TWENTY-FOUR.**</u>

<u>**EVALUATION OF DMSO'S SUITABILITY FOR THE TREATMENT OF SKIN CANCER IN A LABORATORY.**</u>

The benefits of DMSO for the treatment of skin cancer are comparable to those of retinoids, which are compounds found in the skin in most cases. As previously mentioned, DMSO can enter the cell membranes and facilitate the penetration of other motes.

One would presume that DMSO treatment results in cell isolation, perhaps through membrane-intermediated processes. DMSO just functions as a wonderful medium for penetrating tissues of the body to transport hematoxylin, with no impact on the excrescence cell itself.

The combination of DMSO and hematoxylin results in the reduction or elimination of free radical pathology, which is prevalent in advanced cancer cases and also decreases cancer pain.

Any cancer victim who has gone through chemotherapy or radiation treatment will possibly have a problem of hair loss, nausea, blisters at the corners of their lips, a metallic aftertaste in their mouth, dry mouth, and blisters on their lips, etc.

So drinking a little quantity of diluted DMSO will ease or lessen many of these signs and symptoms while patients who have not received chemotherapy or radiation treatment benefit significantly from DMSO intravenous infusions, intramuscular injections, topical operations, and oral application.

<u>DMSO TREATMENT FOR ANIMALS; HORSE AND DOG.</u>

Horses and dogs like every other human have greatly benefited from the use of DMSO as a healing therapy. It is used to treat intracranial hypertension, musculoskeletal disorders, and interstitial cystitis in these animals.

This is made feasible because of the anti-inflammatory agent, cryo-protective and radio-protective properties embedded in DMSO. When these animals are treated with DMSO, although they emit this garlic-like odor, however, the solvent improves the animal's skin and also helps the tissues of the skin absorb other medications rapidly.

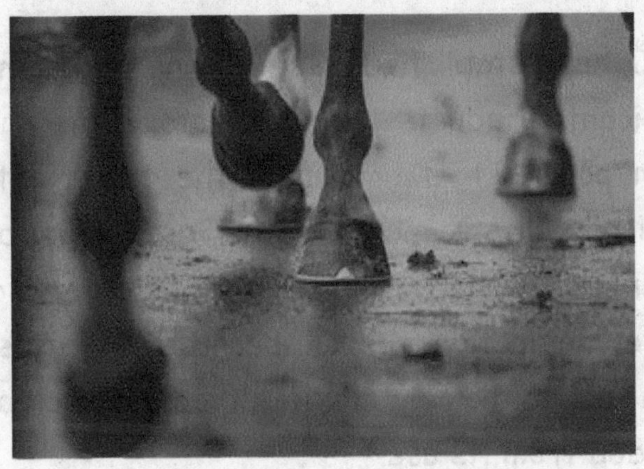

However, it is not advisable to administer DMSO to pregnant animals or hypertensive animals with liver diseases.

Treatment Strategy.

* Topically rub 10 grams of DMSO solution on the affected animal every 6 hours daily for 2 weeks (14 days).

* Visit the veterinarian if symptoms continue after administering DMSO for the state number of days.

CONCLUSION.

DMSO has established itself as one of the most significant products in the history of easing human pains. It is helpful in the treatment of practically all disorders whether used alone or in combination with other drugs and has proven to be a safe medication for all because no cases of death or extremely toxic effects have been recorded from its use.

Its adaptability in use allows it to be used by any medical practice. When an illness is unclear, symptoms may be foggy and tests may be inconclusive. DMSO consistently helps in these conditions.

Medical care is constantly changing. In the early years of the United States, well-known doctors would subject their patients to bleeding in other to get rid of bad blood leading to the death of those patients in most cases. Some years back sailors were being mocked by medical experts for using limes, oranges, and lemons to treat scurvy.

They think it's absurd to think that vitamin C can treat a dangerous condition like scurvy, and these seamen weren't classic doctors looking forward; they had no drug knowledge. Not only DMSO, but other treatments like homeopathic as well, have received little attention in the US despite being proven to be secure and efficient.